Keto Chaffle Cooking Guide

Innovative Ways to Cook Chaffles

Imogene Cook

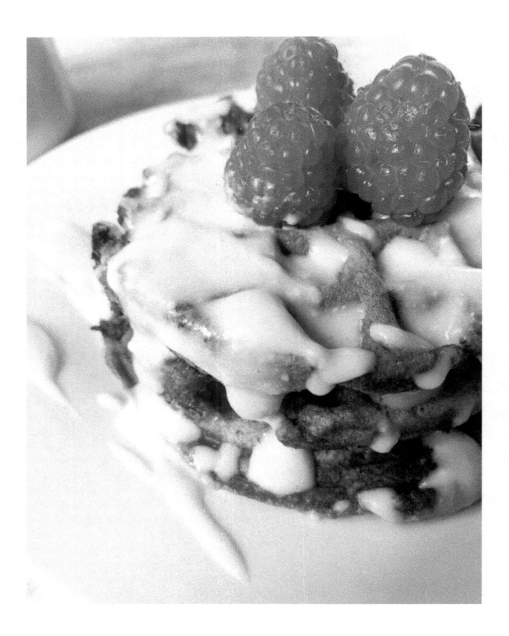

TABLE OF CONTENTS

How to Make Chaffles?

Equipment and Ingredients Discussed

Making chaffles requires five simple steps and nothing more than a waffle maker for flat chaffles and a waffle bowl maker for chaffle bowls.

To make chaffles, you will need two necessary ingredients –eggs and cheese. My preferred cheeses are cheddar cheese or mozzarella cheese. These melt quickly, making them the go-to for most recipes. Meanwhile, always ensure that your cheeses are finely grated or thinly sliced for use.

Now, to make a standard chaffle:

First, preheat your waffle maker until adequately hot.

Meanwhile, in a bowl, mix the egg with cheese on hand until well combined.

Open the iron, pour in a quarter or half of the mixture, and close.

Cook the chaffle for 5 to 7 minutes or until it is crispy.

Transfer the chaffle to a plate and allow cooling before serving.

11 Tips to Make Chaffles

My surefire ways to turn out the crispiest of chaffles:

Preheat Well: Yes! It sounds obvious to preheat the waffle iron before usage. However, preheating the iron moderately

will not get your chaffles as crispy as you will like. The best way to preheat before cooking is to ensure that the iron is very hot.

Not-So-Cheesy: Will you prefer to have your chaffles less cheesy? Then use mozzarella cheese.

Not-So Eggy: If you aren't comfortable with the smell of eggs in your chaffles, try using egg whites instead of egg yolks or whole eggs.

To Shred or to Slice: Many recipes call for shredded cheese when making chaffles, but I find sliced cheeses to offer crispier pieces. While I stick with mostly shredded cheese for convenience's sake, be at ease to use sliced cheese in the same quantity. When using sliced cheeses, arrange two to four pieces in the waffle iron, top with the beaten eggs, and some slices of the cheese. Cover and cook until crispy.

Shallower Irons: For better crisps on your chaffles, use shallower waffle irons as they cook easier and faster.

Layering: Don't fill up the waffle iron with too much batter. Work between a quarter and a half cup of total ingredients per batch for correctly done chaffles.

Patience: It is a virtue even when making chaffles. For the best results, allow the chaffles to sit in the iron for 5 to 7 minutes before serving.

No Peeking: 7 minutes isn't too much of a time to wait for the outcome of your chaffles, in my opinion.

Opening the iron and checking on the chaffle before

it is done stands you a worse chance of ruining it.

Crispy Cooling: For better crisp, I find that allowing the chaffles to cool further after they are transferred to a plate aids a lot.

Easy Cleaning: For the best cleanup, wet a paper towel and wipe the inner parts of the iron clean while still warm. Kindly note that the iron should be warm but not hot!

Brush It: Also, use a clean toothbrush to clean between the iron's teeth for a thorough cleanup. You may also use a dry, rough sponge to clean the iron while it is still warm.

Egg & Chives Chaffle Sandwich Roll

Preparation time: 10 minutes

Cooking Time: 0 Minute

Servings: 2

Ingredients:

- 2 tablespoons mayonnaise
- 1 hard-boiled egg, chopped
- 1 tablespoon chives, chopped
- 2 basic chaffles

Directions:

1. In a bowl, mix the mayo, egg and chives.
2. Spread the mixture on top of the chaffles.
3. Roll the chaffle.

Nutrition:

Calories 258 Total Fat 12g Saturated Fat 2.8g Cholesterol 171mg Sodium 271mg Potassium 71mg Total Carbohydrate 7.5g Dietary Fiber 0.1g Protein 5.9g Total Sugars 2.3g

Basic Chaffles Recipe for Sandwiches

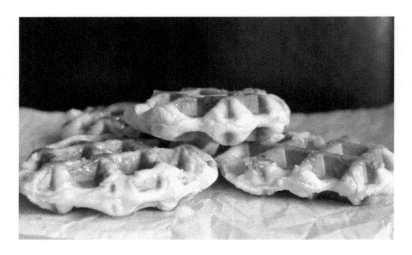

Servings:2

Cooking Time: 5 Minutes

Ingredients:

- 1/2 cup mozzarella cheese, shredded
- 1 large egg
- 2 tbsps. Almond flour
- 1/2 tsp psyllium husk powder
- 1/4 tsp baking powder

Directions:

1. Grease your Belgian waffle maker with cooking spray.
2. Beat the egg with a fork; once the egg is beaten, add almond flour, husk powder, and baking powder.
3. Add cheese to the egg mixture and mix until combined.
4. Pour batter in the center of Belgian waffle and close the lid.
5. Cook chaffles for about 2-3 minutes Utes until well cooked.
6. Carefully transfer the chaffles to plate.
7. The chaffles are perfect for a sandwich base.

Nutrition:

Protein: 29% 60 kcal Fat: 63% 132 kcal Carbohydrates: 18 kcal

Cereal Chaffle Cake

Preparation time: 10 minutes

Cooking Time: 8 Minutes

Servings: 3

Ingredients:

- 1 egg
- 2 tablespoons almond flour
- ½ teaspoon coconut flour
- 1 tablespoon melted butter
- 1 tablespoon cream cheese
- 1 tablespoon plain cereal, crushed
- ¼ teaspoon vanilla extract
- ¼ teaspoon baking powder
- 1 tablespoon sweetener
- 1/8 teaspoon xanthan gum

Directions:

1. Plug in your waffle maker to preheat.
2. Add all the ingredients in a large bowl.

3. Mix until well blended.

4. Let the batter rest for 2 minutes before cooking.

5. Pour half of the mixture into the waffle maker.

6. Seal and cook for 4 minutes.

7. Make the next chaffle using the same steps.

Nutrition:

Calories154 Total Fat 21.2g Saturated Fat 10 g Cholesterol 113.3mg Sodium 96.9mg Potassium 453 mg Total Carbohydrate 5.9g Dietary Fiber 1.7g Protein 4.6g Total Sugars 2.7g

Asian Chaffles

Preparation time: 9 minutes

Cooking Time: 28 Minutes

Servings: 4

Ingredients:

For the chaffles:

- 2 eggs, beaten
- 1 cup finely grated mozzarella cheese
- ½ tsp baking powder
- ¼ cup shredded radishes

For the sauce:

- 2 tsp coconut aminos
- 2 tbsp sugar-free ketchup
- 1 tbsp sugar-free maple syrup
- 2 tsp Worcestershire sauce

For the topping:

- 1 tbsp mayonnaise
- 2 tbsp chopped fresh scallions

- 2 tbsp bonito flakes
- 1 tsp dried seaweed powder
- 1 tbsp pickled ginger

Directions:

For the chaffles:

1. Preheat the waffle iron.
2. In a medium bowl, mix the eggs, mozzarella cheese, baking powder, and radishes.
3. Open the iron and add a quarter of the mixture. Close and cook until crispy, 7 minutes.
4. Transfer the chaffle to a plate and make a 3 more chaffles in the same manner.

For the sauce:

5. Combine the coconut aminos, ketchup, maple syrup, and Worcestershire sauce in a medium bowl and mix well.

For the topping:

6. In another mixing bowl, mix the mayonnaise, scallions, bonito flakes, seaweed powder, and ginger.

To Servings:

7. Arrange the chaffles on four different plates and swirl the sauce on top. Spread the topping on the chaffles and serve afterward.

Nutrition:

Calories 90 Fats 3.32g Carbs 2.97g Net Carbs 2.17g Protein 09g

Bacon & Chicken Ranch Chaffle

Preparation time: 10 minutes

Cooking Time: 8 Minutes

Servings: 4

Ingredients:

- 1 egg
- ¼ cup chicken cubes, cooked
- 1 slice bacon, cooked and chopped
- ¼ cup cheddar cheese, shredded
- 1 teaspoon ranch dressing powder

Directions:

1. Preheat your waffle maker.
2. In a bowl, mix all the ingredients.
3. Add half of the mixture to your waffle maker.
4. Cover and cook for minutes.
5. Make the second chaffle using the same steps.

Nutrition:

Calories 200Total Fat 14 g Saturated Fat g Cholesterol 129 mg Sodium 463 mg Potassium 130 mg Total Carbohydrate 2 g Dietary Fiber 1 g Protein 16 g Total Sugars 1 g

Keto Cocoa Chaffles

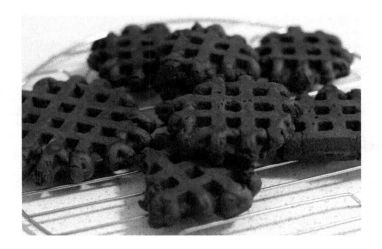

Servings:2

Cooking Time: 5 Minutes

Ingredients:

- 1 large egg
- 1/2 cup shredded cheddar cheese
- 1 tbsp. cocoa powder
- 2 tbsps. almond flour

Directions:

1. Preheat your round waffle maker on medium-high heat.
2. Mix together egg, cheese, almond flour, cocoa powder and vanilla in a small mixing bowl.

3. Pour chaffles mixture into the center of the waffle iron.

4. Close the waffle maker and let cook for 3-5 minutes Utes or until waffle is golden brown and set.

5. Carefully remove chaffles from the waffle maker.

6. Serve hot and enjoy!

Nutrition:

Protein: 20% 49 kcal Fat: % 183 kcal Carbohydrates: 7% 17 kcal

Barbecue Chaffle

Preparation time: 10 minutes

Cooking Time: 8 Minutes

Servings: 2

Ingredients:

- 1 egg, beaten
- ½ cup cheddar cheese, shredded
- ½ teaspoon barbecue sauce
- ¼ teaspoon baking powder

Directions:

1. Plug in your waffle maker to preheat.
2. Mix all the ingredients in a bowl.
3. Pour half of the mixture to your waffle maker.
4. Cover and cook for minutes.
5. Repeat the same steps for the next barbecue chaffle.

Nutrition:

Calories 295 Total Fat 23 g Saturated Fat 13 g Cholesterol 223 mg Sodium 414 mg Potassium 179 mg Total Carbohydrate 2 g Dietary Fiber 1 g Protein 20 g Total Sugars 1 g

Chicken And Chaffle Nachos

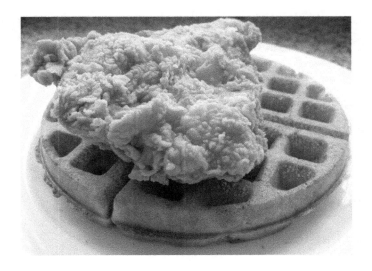

Preparation time: 20 minutes

Cooking Time: 33 Minutes

Servings: 5

Ingredients:

For the chaffles:

- 2 eggs, beaten
- 1 cup finely grated Mexican cheese blend

For the chicken-cheese topping:

- 2 tbsp butter

- 1 tbsp almond flour
- ¼ cup unsweetened almond milk
- 1 cup finely grated cheddar cheese + more to garnish
- 3 bacon slices, cooked and chopped
- 2 cups cooked and diced chicken breasts
- 2 tbsp hot sauce
- 2 tbsp chopped fresh scallions

Directions:

For the chaffles:

1. Preheat the waffle iron.
2. In a medium bowl, mix the eggs and Mexican cheese blend.
3. Open the iron and add a quarter of the mixture. Close and cook until crispy, 7 minutes.
4. Transfer the chaffle to a plate and make 3 more chaffles in the same manner.
5. Place the chaffles on serving plates and set aside for serving.

For the chicken-cheese topping:

6. Melt the butter in a large skillet and mix in the almond flour until brown, 1 minute.

7. Pour the almond milk and whisk until well combined. Simmer until thickened, 2 minutes.

8. Stir in the cheese to melt, 2 minutes and then mix in the bacon, chicken, and hot sauce.

9. Spoon the mixture onto the chaffles and top with some more cheddar cheese.

10. Garnish with the scallions and serve immediately.

Nutrition:

Calories 524 Fats 37.51g Carbs 3.55g Net Carbs 3.25g Protein 41.86g

Ham, Cheese & Tomato Chaffle Sandwich

Preparation time: 10 minutes

Cooking Time: 10 Minutes

Servings: 4

Ingredients:

- 1 teaspoon olive oil
- 2 slices ham
- 4 basic chaffles
- 1 tablespoon mayonnaise
- 2 slices Provolone cheese
- 1 tomato, sliced

Directions:

1. Add the olive oil to a pan over medium heat.
2. Cook the ham for 1 minute per side.
3. Spread the chaffles with mayonnaise.
4. Top with the ham, cheese and tomatoes

5. Top with another chaffle to make a sandwich.

Nutrition:

Calories 198 Total Fat 14.7g Saturated Fat 3g Cholesterol 37mg Sodium 664mg Total Carbohydrate 4.6g Dietary Fiber 0.7g Total Sugars 1.5g Protein 12.2g Potassium 193mg

Simple Savory Chaffle

Preparation Time: 10 minutes

Servings:4

Cooking Time: 7–9 Minutes

Ingredients:

Batter

- 4 eggs
- 1 cup grated mozzarella cheese
- 1 cup grated provolone cheese
- ½ cup almond flour
- 2 tablespoons coconut flour
- 2½ teaspoons baking powder
- Salt and pepper to taste

Other

- 2 tablespoons butter to brush the waffle maker

Directions:

1. Preheat the waffle maker.
2. Add the grated mozzarella and provolone cheese to a bowl and mix.
3. Add the almond and coconut flour and baking powder and season with salt and pepper.
4. Mix with a wire whisk and crack in the eggs.
5. Stir everything together until batter forms.
6. Brush the heated waffle maker with butter and add a few tablespoons of the batter.
7. Close the lid and cook for about 8 minutes depending on your waffle maker.
8. Serve and enjoy.

Nutrition:

Calories 352, fat 27.2 g, carbs 8.3 g, sugar 0.5 g, Protein 15 g, sodium 442 mg

Pizza Chaffle

Preparation Time: 10 minutes

Servings:4

Cooking Time:7–9 Minutes

Ingredients:

Batter

- 4 eggs
- 1½ cups grated mozzarella cheese
- ½ cup grated parmesan cheese
- 2 tablespoons tomato sauce
- ¼ cup almond flour
- 1½ teaspoons baking powder
- Salt and pepper to taste
- 1 teaspoon dried oregano
- ¼ cup sliced salami

Other

- 2 tablespoons olive oil for brushing the waffle maker
- ¼ cup tomato sauce for serving
-

Directions:

1. Preheat the waffle maker.
2. Add the grated mozzarella and grated parmesan to a bowl and mix.
3. Add the almond flour and baking powder and season with salt and pepper and dried oregano.
4. Mix with a wooden spoon or wire whisk and crack in the eggs.
5. Stir everything together until batter forms.
6. Stir in the chopped salami.
7. Brush the heated waffle maker with olive oil and add a few tablespoons of the batter.
8. Close the lid and cook for about 7–minutes depending on your waffle maker.
9. Serve with extra tomato sauce on top and enjoy.

Nutrition:

Calories 319, fat 25.2 g, carbs 5.9 g, sugar 1.7 g, Protein 19.3 g, sodium 596 mg

Bacon Chaffle

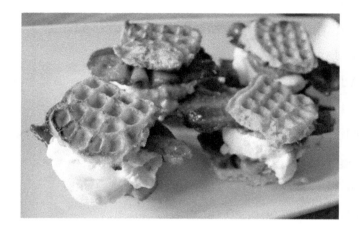

Preparation Time: 10 minutes

Servings:4

Cooking Time:7–9 Minutes

Ingredients:

Batter

- 4 eggs
- 2 cups shredded mozzarella
- 2 ounces finely chopped bacon
- Salt and pepper to taste
- 1 teaspoon dried oregano
-

Other

- 2 tablespoons olive oil for brushing the waffle maker

Directions:

1. Preheat the waffle maker.
2. Crack the eggs into a bowl and add the grated mozzarella cheese.
3. Mix until just combined and stir in the chopped bacon.
4. Season with salt and pepper and dried oregano.
5. Brush the heated waffle maker with olive oil and add a few tablespoons of the batter.
6. Close the lid and cook for about 7–8 minutes depending on your waffle maker.

Nutrition:

Calories 241, fat 19.8 g, carbs 1.3 g, sugar 0.4 g, Protein 14.8 g, sodium 4 mg

Chaffles Breakfast Bowl

Preparation Time: 10 minutes

Servings:2

Cooking Time: 5 Minutes

Ingredients:

- 1 egg
- 1/2 cup cheddar cheese shredded
- pinch of Italian seasoning
- 1 tbsp. pizza sauce

TOPPING

- 1/2 avocado sliced
- 2 eggs boiled
- 1 tomato, halves
- 4 oz. fresh spinach leaves

Directions:

1. Preheat your waffle maker and grease with cooking spray.
2. Crack an egg in a small bowl and beat with Italian seasoning and pizza sauce.

3. Add shredded cheese to the egg and spices mixture.
4. Pour 1 tbsp. shredded cheese in a waffle maker and cook for 30 sec.
5. Pour Chaffles batter in the waffle maker and close the lid.
6. Cook chaffles for about 4 minutes Utes until crispy and brown.
7. Carefully remove chaffles from the maker.
8. Serve on the bed of spinach with boil egg, avocado slice, and tomatoes.
9. Enjoy!

Nutrition:

Protein: 23% 77 kcal Fat: 66% 222 kcal Carbohydrates: 11% 39 kcal

Morning Chaffles With Berries

Preparation Time: 10 minutes

Servings: 4

Cooking Time: 5 Minutes

Ingredients:

- 1 cup egg whites
- 1 cup cheddar cheese, shredded
- ¼ cup almond flour
- ¼ cup heavy cream

TOPPING

- 4 oz. raspberries
- 4 oz. strawberries.
- 1 oz. keto chocolate flakes
- 1 oz. feta cheese.

Directions:

1. Preheat your square waffle maker and grease with cooking spray.
2. Beat egg white in a small bowl with flour.
3. Add shredded cheese to the egg whites and flour mixture and mix well.
4. Add cream and cheese to the egg mixture.
5. Pour Chaffles batter in a waffle maker and close the lid.
6. Cook chaffles for about 4 minutes Utes until crispy and brown.
7. Carefully remove chaffles from the maker.
8. Serve with berries, cheese, and chocolate on top.
9. Enjoy!

Nutrition:

Protein: 28% 68 kcal Fat: 67% 163 kcal Carbohydrates: 5% 12 kcal

Chicken Bites with Chaffles

Preparation time: 10 minutes

Cooking Time: 10 minutes

Servings: 2

Ingredients:

- 1 chicken breasts cut into 2x2 inch chunks
- 1 egg, whisked
- 1/4 cup almond flour
- 2 tbsps. onion powder
- 2 tbsps. garlic powder
- 1 tsp. dried oregano
- 1 tsp. paprika powder
- 1 tsp. salt
- 1/2 tsp. black pepper
- 2 tbsps. avocado oil

Directions:

1. Add all the dry ingredients together into a large bowl. Mix well.

2. Place the eggs into a separate bowl.
3. Dip each chicken piece into the egg and then into the dry ingredients.
4. Heat oil in 10-inch skillet, add oil.
5. Once avocado oil is hot, place the coated chicken nuggets onto a skillet and cook for 6-8 minutes Utes until cooked and golden brown.
6. Serve with chaffles and raspberries.
7. Enjoy!

Nutrition:

Total Calories 401 kcal Fats 219 g Protein 32.35 g Nectars 1.46 g Fiber 3 g

Crunchy Fish and Chaffle Bites

Servings:4

Cooking Time: 15 Minutes

Ingredients:

- 1 lb. cod fillets, sliced into 4 slices
- 1 tsp. sea salt
- 1 tsp. garlic powder
- 1 egg, whisked
- 1 cup almond flour
- 2 tbsp. avocado oil

CHAFFLE Ingredients:

- 2 eggs
- 1/2 cup cheddar cheese
- 2 tbsps. almond flour
- ½ tsp. Italian seasoning

Directions:

1. Mix together chaffle ingredients in a bowl and make 4 square

2. Put the chaffles in a preheated chaffle maker.

3. Mix together the salt, pepper, and garlic powder in a mixing bowl. Toss the cod cubes in this mixture and let sit for 10 minutes Utes.

4. Then dip each cod slice into the egg mixture and then into the almond flour.

5. Heat oil in skillet and fish cubes for about 2-3 minutes Utes, until cooked and browned

6. Serve on chaffles and enjoy!

Nutrition:

Protein: 38% 121 kcal Fat: 59% 189 kcal Carbohydrates: 3% 11 kcal

Grill Pork Chaffle Sandwich

Preparation time: 10 minutes

Servings:2

Cooking Time: 15 Minutes

Ingredients:

- 1/2 cup mozzarella, shredded
- 1 egg
- I pinch garlic powder

PORK PATTY

- 1/2 cup pork, minutes
- 1 tbsp. green onion, diced
- 1/2 tsp Italian seasoning
- Lettuce leaves

Directions:

1. Preheat the square waffle maker and grease with
2. Mix together egg, cheese and garlic powder in a small mixing bowl.

3. Pour batter in a preheated waffle maker and close the lid.

4. Make 2 chaffles from this batter.

5. Cook chaffles for about 2-3 minutes Utes until cooked through.

6. Meanwhile, mix together pork patty ingredients in a bowl and make 1 large patty.

7. Grill pork patty in a preheated grill for about 3-4 minutes Utes per side until cooked through.

8. Arrange pork patty between two chaffles with lettuce leaves. Cut sandwich to make a triangular sandwich.

9. Enjoy!

Nutrition:

Protein: 48% 85 kcal Fat: 48% 86 kcal Carbohydrates: 4% 7 kcal

Chaffle & Chicken Lunch Plate

Preparation time: 10 minutes

Servings:2

Cooking Time: 15 Minutes

Ingredients:

- 1 large egg
- 1/2 cup jack cheese, shredded
- 1 pinch salt

For Serving

- 1 chicken leg
- salt
- pepper
- 1 tsp. garlic, minutes
- 1 egg
- I tsp avocado oil

Directions:

1. Heat your square waffle maker and grease with cooking spray.
2. Pour Chaffle batter into the skillet and cook for about 3 minutes Utes.
3. Meanwhile, heat oil in a pan, over medium heat.
4. Once the oil is hot, add chicken thigh and garlic then, cook for about 5 minutes Utes. Flip and cook for another 3-4 minutes.
5. Season with salt and pepper and give them a good mix.
6. Transfer cooked thigh to plate.
7. Fry the egg in the same pan for about 1-2 minutes Utes according to your choice.
8. Once chaffles are cooked, serve with fried egg and chicken thigh.
9. Enjoy!

Nutrition:

Protein: 31% 138 kcal Fat: 66% 292 kcal Carbohydrates: 2% kcal

Chaffle Egg Sandwich

Preparation time: 10 minutes

Cooking Time: 10 Minutes

Servings:2

Ingredients:

- 2 minutes keto chaffle
- 2 slice cheddar cheese
- 1 egg simple omelet

Directions:

1. Prepare your oven on 4000 F.
2. Arrange egg omelet and cheese slice between chaffles.
3. Bake in the preheated oven for about 4-5 minutes Utes until cheese is melted.
4. Once the cheese is melted, remove from the oven.
5. Serve and enjoy!

Nutrition:

Protein: 29% 144 kcal Fat: % 337 kcal Carbohydrates: 3% 14 kcal

Chaffle Minutes Sandwich

Preparation time: 10 minutes

Cooking Time: 10 Minutes

Servings:2

Ingredients:

- 1 large egg
- 1/8 cup almond flour
- 1/2 tsp. garlic powder
- 3/4 tsp. baking powder
- 1/2 cup shredded cheese

SANDWICH FILLING

- 2 slices deli ham
- 2 slices tomatoes
- 1 slice cheddar cheese

Directions:

1. Grease your square waffle maker and preheat it on medium heat.
2. Mix together chaffle ingredients in a mixing bowl until well combined.
3. Pour batter into a square waffle and make two chaffles.
4. Once chaffles are cooked, remove from the maker.
5. For a sandwich, arrange deli ham, tomato slice and cheddar cheese between two chaffles.
6. Cut sandwich from the center.
7. Serve and enjoy!

Nutrition:

Protein: 29% 70 kcal Fat: 66% 159 kcal Carbohydrates: 4% 10 kcal

Chaffle Cheese Sandwich

Preparation time: 10 minutes

Servings: 1

Cooking Time: 10 Minutes

Ingredients:

- 2 square keto chaffle
- 2 slice cheddar cheese
- 2 lettuce leaves

Directions:

1. Prepare your oven on 4000 F.
2. Arrange lettuce leave and cheese slice between chaffles.
3. Bake in the preheated oven for about 4-5 minutes Utes until cheese is melted.
4. Once the cheese is melted, remove from the oven.
5. Serve and enjoy!

Nutrition:

Protein: 28% kcal Fat: 69% 149 kcal Carbohydrates: 3% 6 kcal

Chicken Zinger Chaffle

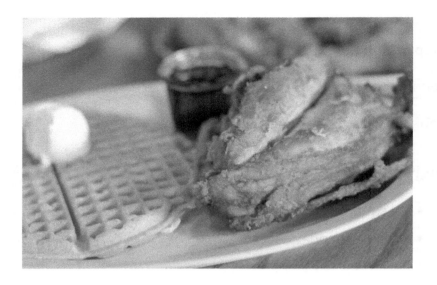

Preparation time: 10 minutes

Servings:2

Cooking Time: 15 Minutes

Ingredients:

- 1 chicken breast, cut into 2 pieces
- 1/2 cup coconut flour
- 1/4 cup finely grated Parmesan
- 1 tsp. paprika
- 1/2 tsp. garlic powder
- 1/2 tsp. onion powder

- 1 tsp. salt& pepper
- 1 egg beaten
- Avocado oil for frying
- Lettuce leaves
- BBQ sauce

CHAFFLE Ingredients:

- 4 oz. cheese
- 2 whole eggs
- 2 oz. almond flour
- 1/4 cup almond flour
- 1 tsp baking powder

Directions:

1. Mix together chaffle ingredients in a bowl.
2. Pour the chaffle batter in preheated greased square chaffle maker.
3. Cook chaffles for about 2-minutesutes until cooked through.
4. Make square chaffles from this batter.
5. Meanwhile mix together coconut flour, parmesan, paprika, garlic powder, onion powder salt and pepper in a bowl.

6. Dip chicken first in coconut flour mixture then in beaten egg.
7. Heat avocado oil in a skillet and cook chicken from both sides. until lightly brown and cooked
8. Set chicken zinger between two chaffles with lettuce and BBQ sauce.
9. Enjoy!

Nutrition:

Protein: 30% 219 kcal Fat: 60% 435 kcal Carbohydrates: 9% 66 kcal

Double Chicken Chaffles

Preparation time: 10 minutes

Servings:2

Cooking Time: 5 Minutes

Ingredients:

- 1/2 cup boil shredded chicken
- 1/4 cup cheddar cheese
- 1/8 cup parmesan cheese
- 1 egg
- 1 tsp. Italian seasoning
- 1/8 tsp. garlic powder
- 1 tsp. cream cheese

Directions:

1. Preheat the Belgian waffle maker.
2. Mix together in chaffle ingredients in a bowl and mix together.
3. Sprinkle 1 tbsp. of cheese in a waffle maker and pour in chaffle batter.
4. Pour 1 tbsp. of cheese over batter and close the lid.

5. Cook chaffles for about 4 to minutes Utes.

6. Serve with a chicken zinger and enjoy the double chicken flavor.

Nutrition:

Protein: 30% 60 kcal Fat: 65% 129 kcal Carbohydrates: 5% 9 kcal

Chaffles With Topping

Preparation time: 10 minutes

Cooking Time: 10 Minutes

Ingredients:

- 1 large egg
- 1 tbsp. almond flour
- 1 tbsp. full-fat Greek yogurt
- 1/8 tsp baking powder
- 1/4 cup shredded Swiss cheese

TOPPING

- 4oz. grill prawns
- 4 oz. steamed cauliflower mash
- 1/2 zucchini sliced
- 3 lettuce leaves
- 1 tomato, sliced
- 1 tbsp. flax seeds

Directions:

1. Make 3 chaffles with the given chaffles ingredients.
2. For serving, arrange lettuce leaves on each chaffle.
3. Top with zucchini slice, grill prawns, cauliflower mash and a tomato slice.
4. Drizzle flax seeds on top.
5. Serve and enjoy

Chaffle With Cheese & Bacon

Preparation time: 10 minutes

Servings:2

Cooking Time: 15 Minutes

Ingredients:

- 1 egg
- 1/2 cup cheddar cheese, shredded
- 1 tbsp. parmesan cheese
- 3/4 tsp coconut flour
- 1/4 tsp baking powder
- 1/8 tsp Italian Seasoning
- pinch of salt
- 1/4 tsp garlic powder

FOR TOPPING

- 1 bacon sliced, cooked and chopped
- 1/2 cup mozzarella cheese, shredded
- 1/4 tsp parsley, chopped

Directions:

1. Preheat oven to 400 degrees.
2. Switch on your minutes waffle maker and grease with cooking spray.
3. Mix together chaffle ingredients in a mixing bowl until combined.
4. Spoon half of the batter in the center of the waffle maker and close the lid. Cook chaffles for about 3-minutesutes until cooked.
5. Carefully remove chaffles from the maker.
6. Arrange chaffles in a greased baking tray.
7. Top with mozzarella cheese, chopped bacon and parsley.
8. And bake in the oven for 4 -5 minutes Utes.
9. Once the cheese is melted, remove from the oven.
10. Serve and enjoy!

Nutrition:

Protein: 28% 90 kcal Fat: 69% 222 kcal Carbohydrates: 3% kcal

Grill Beefsteak and Chaffle

Preparation time: 10 minutes

Servings: 1

Cooking Time: 10 Minutes

Ingredients:

- 1 beefsteak rib eye
- 1 tsp salt
- 1 tsp pepper
- 1 tbsp. lime juice
- 1 tsp garlic

Directions:

1. Prepare your grill for direct heat.
2. Mix together all spices and rub over beefsteak evenly.
3. Place the beef on the grill rack over medium heat.
4. Cover and cook steak for about6 to 8 minutes Utes. Flip and cook for another 5 minutes Utes until cooked through.
5. Serve with keto simple chaffle and enjoy!

Nutrition:

Protein: 51% 274 kcal Fat: 45% 243 kcal Carbohydrates: 4% 22 kcal

Cauliflower Chaffles And Tomatoes

Preparation time: 10 minutes

Servings:2

Cooking Time: 15 Minutes

Ingredients:

- 1/2 cup cauliflower
- 1/4 tsp. garlic powder
- 1/4 tsp. black pepper
- 1/4 tsp. Salt
- 1/2 cup shredded cheddar cheese
- 1 egg

FOR TOPPING

- 1 lettuce leave
- 1 tomato sliced
- 4 oz. cauliflower steamed, mashed
- 1 tsp sesame seeds

Directions:

1. Add all chaffle ingredients into a blender and mix well.
2. Sprinkle 1/8 shredded cheese on the waffle maker and pour cauliflower mixture in a preheated waffle maker and sprinkle the rest of the cheese over it.
3. Cook chaffles for about 4-5 minutes Utes until cooked
4. For serving, lay lettuce leaves over chaffle top with steamed cauliflower and tomato.
5. Drizzle sesame seeds on top.
6. Enjoy!

Nutrition:

Protein: 25% 49 kcal Fat: 65% 128 kcal Carbohydrates: 10% 21 kcal

Carrot Chaffles

Servings: 6

Cooking Time: 18 Minutes

Ingredients:

- ¾ cup almond flour
- 1 tablespoon walnuts, chopped
- 2 tablespoons powdered Erythritol
- 1 teaspoon organic baking powder
- ½ teaspoon ground cinnamon
- ½ teaspoon pumpkin pie spice
- 1 organic egg, beaten
- 2 tablespoons heavy whipping cream
- 2 tablespoons butter, melted
- ½ cup carrot, peeled and shredded

Directions:

1. Preheat a mini waffle iron and then grease it.
2. In a bowl, place the flour, walnut, Erythritol, cinnamon, baking powder and spices and mix well.

3. Add the egg, heavy whipping cream and butter and mix until well combined.
4. Gently, fold in the carrot.
5. Add about 3 tablespoons of the mixture into preheated waffle iron and cook for about 2½-3 minutes or until golden brown.
6. Repeat with the remaining mixture.
7. Serve warm.

Nutrition:

Calories:165 Net Carb:2.4g Fat:14.7g Saturated Fat:4.4g Carbohydrates: 4.4g Dietary Fiber: 2g Sugar: 1g Protein: 1.5g

Yogurt Chaffles

Servings: 3

Cooking Time: 10 Minutes

Ingredients:

- ½ cup shredded mozzarella
- 1 egg
- 2 Tbsp ground almonds
- ½ tsp psyllium husk
- ¼ tsp baking powder
- 1 Tbsp yogurt

Directions:

1. Turn on waffle maker to heat and oil it with cooking spray.
2. Whisk eggs in a bowl.
3. Add in remaining ingredients except mozzarella and mix well.
4. Add mozzarella and mix once again. Let it sit for 5 minutes.
5. Add ⅓ cup batter into each waffle mold.

6. Close and cook for 4-5 minutes.

7. Repeat with remaining batter.

Nutrition:

Carbs: 2 g ; Fat: 5 g ;Protein: 4 g ;Calories: 93

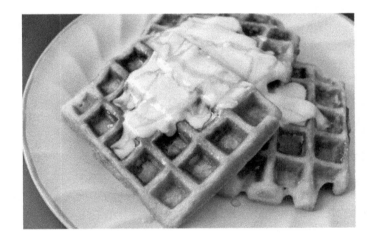

Chocolate Peanut Butter Chaffles

Preparation time: 5 minutes

Cooking Time: 8 Minutes

Servings: 2

Ingredients:

- 1 organic egg, beaten
- ¼ cup mozzarella cheese, shredded
- 2 tablespoons creamy peanut butter
- 1 tablespoon almond flour
- 1 tablespoon granulated erythritol
- 1 teaspoon organic vanilla extract
- 1 tablespoon 70% dark chocolate chips

Directions:

1. Preheat a mini waffle iron and then grease it.
2. In a bowl, add all ingredients except chocolate and beat until well combined. Gently, fold in the chocolate chips.
3. Place half of the mixture into preheated waffle iron and cook for about 4 minutes.

4. Repeat with the remaining mixture.

5. Serve warm.

Nutrition:

Calories 214 Net Carbs 4.1 g Total Fat 18 g Saturated Fat 5.4 g Cholesterol 84 mg Sodium 128 mg Total Carbs 6.4 g Fiber 2.3 g Sugar 2.1 g Protein 8.8 g

Ube Chaffles With Ice Cream

Preparation time: 5 minutes

Cooking Time: 10 Minutes

Servings: 2

Ingredients:

- 1/3 cup mozzarella cheese, shredded
- 1 tbsp whipped cream cheese
- 2 tbsp sweetener
- 1 egg
- 2-3 drops ube or pandan extract
- 1/2 tsp baking powder
- Keto ice cream

Directions:

1. Add in 2 or 3 drops of ube extract, mix until creamy and smooth.
2. Pour half of the batter mixture in the mini waffle maker and cook for about 5 minutes.
3. Repeat the same steps with the remaining batter mixture.

4. Top with keto ice cream and enjoy.

Nutrition:

Calories per Preparation time: 5 minutes 65Kcal ; Fats: 16 g ;
Carbs: 7 g ; Protein: 22 g

2- Berries Chaffles

Preparation time: 5 minutes

Cooking Time: 10 Minutes

Servings: 2

Ingredients:

- 1 organic egg
- 1 teaspoon organic vanilla extract
- 1 tablespoon of almond flour
- 1 teaspoon organic baking powder
- Pinch of ground cinnamon
- 1 cup Mozzarella cheese, shredded
- 2 tablespoons fresh blueberries
- 2 tablespoons fresh blackberries

Directions:

1. Preheat a waffle iron and then grease it.
2. In a bowl, place thee egg and vanilla extract and beat well.
3. Add the flour, baking powder and cinnamon and mix well.

4. Add the Mozzarella cheese and mix until just combined.

5. Gently, fold in the berries.

6. Place half of the mixture into preheated waffle iron and cook for about 4-5 minutes or until golden brown.

7. Repeat with the remaining mixture.

8. Serve warm.

Nutrition:

Calories:112   Net   Carb:3.8g   Fat:6.7g   Saturate   Fat:2.3g Carbohydrates: 5g Dietary Fiber: 1.2g Sugar: 1. Protein: 7g

Cinnamon Swirl Chaffles

Servings: 3

Cooking Time: 12 Minutes

Ingredients:

For Chaffles:

- 1 organic egg
- ½ cup Mozzarella cheese, shredded
- 1 tablespoon almond flour
- ¼ teaspoon organic baking powder
- 1 teaspoon granulated Erythritol
- 1 teaspoon ground cinnamon

For Topping:

- 1 tablespoon butter
- 1 teaspoon ground cinnamon
- 2 teaspoons powdered Erythritol

Directions:

1. Preheat a waffle iron and then grease it.
2. For chaffles: in a bowl, place all ingredients and mix until well combined.

For topping:

3. In a small microwave-safe bowl, place all ingredients and microwave for about 15 seconds.
4. Remove from microwave and mix well.
5. Place 1/3 of the chaffles mixture into preheated waffle iron.
6. Top with 1/3 of the butter mixture and with a skewer, gently swirl into the chaffles mixture.
7. Cook for about 3-4 minutes or until golden brown.
8. Repeat with the remaining chaffles and topping mixture.
9. Serve warm.

Nutrition:

Calories:87 Net Carb:1g Fat: 7.4g   Saturated   Fat:3.5g
Carbohydrates: 2.1g Dietary Fiber: 1.1g Sugar: 0.2g Protein: 3.3g

Chocolate Cream Cheese Chaffles

Preparation time: 5 minutes

Cooking Time: 8 Minutes

Servings: 2

Ingredients:

- 1 large organic egg, beaten
- 1 ounce cream cheese, softened
- 1 tablespoon sugar-free chocolate syrup
- 1 tablespoon Erythritol
- ½ tablespoon cacao powder
- ¼ teaspoon organic baking powder
- ½ teaspoon organic vanilla extract

Directions:

1. Preheat a mini waffle iron and then grease it.
2. In a medium bowl, place all ingredients and with a fork, mix until well combined.

3. Place half of the mixture into preheated waffle iron and cook for about 4 minutes or until golden brown.
4. Repeat with the remaining mixture.
5. Serve warm.

Nutrition:

Calories:103   Net   Carb:4.2g   Fat:7.7g   Saturated   Fat:4.1g Carbohydrates: 4. Dietary Fiber: 0.4g Sugar: 2g Protein: 4.5g

Big Cheese Chaffles

Servings: 1

Cooking Time: 6 Minutes

Ingredients:

- 2 ounces american cheese, sliced thinly in triangles
- 1 large organic egg, beaten

Directions:

1. Preheat a waffle iron and then grease it.
2. Arrange 1 thin layer of cheese slices in the bottom of preheated waffle iron.
3. Place the beaten egg on top of the cheese.
4. Now, arrange another layer of cheese slices on top to cover evenly.
5. Cook for about 6 minutes.
6. Serve warm.

Nutrition:

Calories 292 Net Carbs 2.4 g Total Fat 23 g Saturated Fat 13.6 g Cholesterol 236 mg Sodium 431 mg Total Carbs 2.4 g Fiber 0 g Sugar 0.4 g Protein 18.3 g

Chaffle Birthday Cake

Preparation time: 8 minutes

Cooking Time: 16 Minutes

Servings: 2

Ingredients:

- Butter cream icing

Birthday Cake Chaffle:

- 3 tbsp cream cheese
- 1 tbsp almond flour
- 5 tbsp coconut flour
- 1 tsp baking powder
- 6 eggs
- 2 tbsp birthday cake syrup

Directions:

1. Scoop 3 tbsp of the mixture into your waffle maker. Cook for 4 minutes and set aside.
2. Repeat the process until you have 4 cake chaffles.

3. Just like a normal cake, start assembling your cake by placing one chaffle at the bottom as the base and add a butter cream icing layer. Repeat the same process.
4. Pipe your cake edges with the icing and pile colorful shredded coconut at the center.
5. Once all the layers are completed, top with more icing and shredded coconut sprinkles.
6. Enjoy!

Nutrition:

Calories per Servings: 390 Kcal ; Fats: 35 g ; Carbs: 18.9 g ; Protein: 11 g

Chaffle Churros

Preparation time: 5 minutes

Cooking Time: 5 Minutes

Servings: 2

Ingredients:

- 1 egg
- 1 Tbsp almond flour
- ½ tsp vanilla extract
- 1 tsp cinnamon, divided
- ¼ tsp baking powder
- ½ cup shredded mozzarella
- 1 Tbsp swerve confectioners' sugar substitute
- 1 Tbsp swerve brown sugar substitute
- 1 Tbsp butter, melted

Directions:

1. Turn on waffle maker to heat and oil it with cooking spray.

2. Mix egg, flour, vanilla extract, ½ tsp cinnamon, baking powder, mozzarella, and sugar substitute in a bowl.
3. Place half of the mixture into waffle maker and cook for 5 minutes, or until desired doneness.
4. Remove and place the second half of the batter into the maker.
5. Cut chaffles into strips.
6. Place strips in a bowl and cover with melted butter.
7. Mix brown sugar substitute and the remaining cinnamon in a bowl.
8. Pour sugar mixture over the strips and toss to coat them well.

Nutrition:

Carbs: 5 g ; Fat: 6 g ; Protein: 5 g ; Calories: 76

Strawberry Chaffles

Preparation time: 5 minutes

Cooking Time: 8 Minutes

Servings: 2

Ingredients:

- 1 organic egg, beaten
- ¼ cup Mozzarella cheese, shredded
- 1 tablespoon cream cheese, softened
- ¼ teaspoon organic baking powder
- 1 teaspoon organic strawberry extract
- 2 fresh strawberries, hulled and sliced

Directions:

1. Preheat a mini waffle iron and then grease it.
2. In a bowl, place all ingredients except strawberry slices and beat until well combined.
3. Fold in the strawberry slices.
4. Place half of the mixture into preheated waffle iron and cook for about minutes or until golden brown.

5. Repeat with the remaining mixture.

6. Serve warm.

Nutrition:

Calories:69 Net Carb:1.6g Fat:4.6g Saturated Fat:2.2g Carbohydrates: 1.9g Dietary Fiber: 0.3g Sugar: 1g Protein: 4.2g

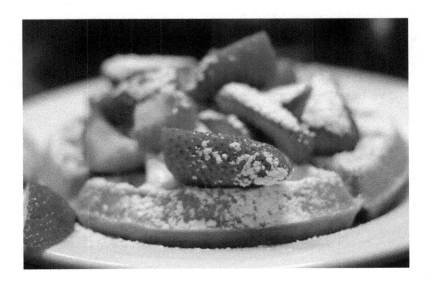

Butter & Cream Cheese Chaffles

Preparation time: 8 minutes

Cooking Time: 16 Minutes

Servings: 2

Ingredients:

- 2 tablespoons butter, melted and cooled
- 2 large organic eggs
- 2 ounces cream cheese, softened
- ¼ cup powdered erythritol
- 1½ teaspoons organic vanilla extract
- Pinch of salt
- ¼ cup almond flour
- 2 tablespoons coconut flour
- 1 teaspoon organic baking powder

Directions:

1. Preheat a mini waffle iron and then grease it.
2. In a bowl, add the butter and eggs and beat until creamy.
3. Add the cream cheese, erythritol, vanilla extract, and salt,

and beat until well combined.

4. Add the flours and baking powder and beat until well combined.

5. Place ¼ of the mixture into preheated waffle iron and cook for about 4 minutes.

6. Repeat with the remaining mixture.

7. Serve warm.

Nutrition:

Calories 217 Net Carbs 3.3 g Total Fat 1g Saturated Fat 8.8 g Cholesterol 124 mg Sodium 173 mg Total Carbs 6.6 g Fiber 3.3 g Sugar 1.2 g Protein 5.3 g

Cinnamon Chaffles

Preparation time: 5 minutes

Cooking Time: 8 Minutes

Servings: 2

Ingredients:

- 1 large organic egg, beaten
- ¾ cup mozzarella cheese, shredded
- ½ tablespoon unsalted butter, melted
- 2 tablespoons blanched almond flour
- 2 tablespoons erythritol
- ½ teaspoon ground cinnamon
- ½ teaspoon Psyllium husk powder
- ¼ teaspoon organic baking powder
- ½ teaspoon organic vanilla extract

Topping

- 1 teaspoon powdered Erythritol
- ¾ teaspoon ground cinnamon

Directions:

1. Preheat a waffle iron and then grease it.
2. For chaffles: In a medium bowl, put all ingredients and with a fork, mix until well combined.
3. Place half of the mixture into preheated waffle iron and cook for about 5 minutes.
4. Repeat with the remaining mixture.
5. Meanwhile, for topping: in a small bowl, mix together the erythritol and cinnamon.
6. Place the chaffles onto serving plates and set aside to cool slightly.
7. Sprinkle with the cinnamon mixture and serve immediately.

Nutrition:

Calories 142 Net Carbs 2.1 g Total Fat 10.6 g Saturated Fat 4 g Cholesterol 106 mg Sodium 122 mg Total Carbs 4.1 g Fiber 2 g Sugar 0.3 g Protein 7.7 g

Glazed Chaffles

Preparation time: 5 minutes

Cooking Time: 5 Minutes

Servings: 2

Ingredients:

- ½ cup mozzarella shredded cheese
- ⅛ cup cream cheese
- 2 Tbsp unflavored whey protein isolate
- 2 Tbsp swerve confectioners' sugar substitute
- ½ tsp baking powder
- ½ tsp vanilla extract
- 1 egg

For the glaze topping:

- 2 Tbsp heavy whipping cream
- 3-4 Tbsp swerve confectioners' sugar substitute ½ tsp vanilla extract

Directions:

1. Turn on waffle maker to heat and oil it with cooking spray.
2. In a microwave-safe bowl, mix mozzarella and cream cheese. Heat at 30 second intervals until melted and fully combined.
3. Add protein, 2 Tbsp sweetener, baking powder to cheese. Knead with hands until well incorporated.
4. Place dough into a mixing bowl and beat in egg and vanilla until a smooth batter forms.
5. Put ⅓ of the batter into waffle maker, and cook for 3-minutes, until golden brown.
6. Repeat until all 3 chaffles are made.
7. Beat glaze ingredients in a bowl and pour over chaffles before serving.

Nutrition:

Carbs: 4 g ; Fat: 6 g ; Protein: 4 g ; Calories: 130

Blueberry Cream Cheese Chaffles

Preparation time: 5 minutes

Cooking Time: 8 Minutes

Servings: 2

Ingredients:

- 1 organic egg, beaten
- 1 tablespoon cream cheese, softened
- 3 tablespoons almond flour
- ¼ teaspoon organic baking powder
- 1 teaspoon organic blueberry extract
- 5-6 fresh blueberries

Directions:

1. Preheat a mini waffle iron and then grease it.
2. In a bowl, place all the ingredients except blueberries and beat until well combined.
3. Fold in the blueberries.
4. Divide the mixture into 5 portions.

5. Place 1 portion of the mixture into preheated waffle iron and cook for about 3-4 minutes or until golden brown.

6. Repeat with the remaining mixture.

7. Serve warm.

Nutrition:

Calories:120   Net   Carb:1.   Fat:9.6g   Saturated   Fat:2.2g Carbohydrates: 3.1g Dietary Fiber: 1.3g Sugar: 1g Protein: 3.2g

Italian Cream Chaffle Sandwich-cake

Preparation time: 8 minutes

Cooking Time: 20 Minutes

Ingredients:

- 4 oz cream cheese, softened, at room temperature
- 4 eggs
- 1 Tbsp melted butter
- 1 tsp vanilla extract
- ½ tsp cinnamon
- 1 Tbsp monk fruit sweetener
- 4 Tbsp coconut flour
- 1 Tbsp almond flour
- 1½ teaspoons baking powder
- 1 Tbsp coconut, shredded and unsweetened
- 1 Tbsp walnuts, chopped

For the Italian cream frosting:

- 2 oz cream cheese, softened, at room temperature
- 2 Tbsp butter room temp

- 2 Tbsp monk fruit sweetener
- ½ tsp vanilla

Directions:

1. Combine cream cheese, eggs, melted butter, vanilla, sweetener, flours, and baking powder in a blender.
2. Add walnuts and coconut to the mixture.
3. Blend to get a creamy mixture.
4. Turn on waffle maker to heat and oil it with cooking spray.
5. Add enough batter to fill waffle maker. Cook for 2-3 minutes, until chaffles are done.
6. Remove and let them cool.
7. Mix all frosting ingredients in another bowl. Stir until smooth and creamy.
8. Frost the chaffles once they have cooled.
9. Top with cream and more nuts.

Nutrition:

Carbs: 31 g ; Fat: 2 g ;Protein: 5 g ; Calories: 168

Whipping Cream Chaffles

Preparation time: 5 minutes

Cooking Time: 8 Minutes

Servings: 2

Ingredients:

- 1 organic egg, beaten
- 1 tablespoon heavy whipping cream
- 2 tablespoons sugar-free peanut butter powder
- 2 tablespoons Erythritol
- ¼ teaspoon organic baking powder
- ¼ teaspoon peanut butter extract

Directions:

1. Preheat a mini waffle iron and then grease it.
2. In a medium bowl, place all ingredients and with a fork, mix until well combined.
3. Place half of the mixture into preheated waffle iron and cook for about 4 minutes or until golden brown.
4. Repeat with the remaining mixture.

5. Serve warm.

Nutrition:

Calories:112 Net Carb:1. Fat:6.9g Saturated Fat:2.7g Carbohydrates: 3.7g Dietary Fiber: 2.1g Sugar: 0.2g Protein: 10.9g

Cinnamon Pumpkin Chaffles

Preparation time: 8 minutes

Cooking Time: 16 Minutes

Servings: 2

Ingredients:

- 2 organic eggs
- 2/3 cup Mozzarella cheese, shredded
- 3 tablespoons sugar-free pumpkin puree
- 3 teaspoons almond flour
- 2 teaspoons granulated Erythritol
- 2 teaspoons ground cinnamon

Directions:

1. Preheat a mini waffle iron and then grease it.
2. In a medium bowl, place all ingredients and with a fork, mix until well combined.
3. Place half of the mixture into preheated waffle iron and cook for about 4 minutes or until golden brown.
4. Repeat with the remaining mixture.

5. Serve warm.

Nutrition:

Calories: Net Carb: 1.4g Fat: 4g Saturated Fat: 1.3g Carbohydrates:2.5g Dietary Fiber: 1.1g Sugar: 0.6g Protein: 4.3g

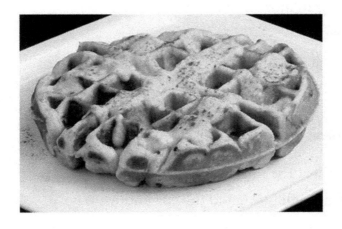

Keto Tuna Melt Chaffle Recipe

Preparation time: 15 minutes

Cooking time: 8 minutes

Servings: 2

Ingredients:

- 1 packet Tuna 2.6 oz with no water
- 1/2 cup mozzarella cheese
- 1 egg
- pinch salt

Directions:

1. Preheat the mini waffle maker
2. In a small bowl, add the egg and whip it up.
3. Add the tuna, cheese, and salt and mix well.
4. Optional step for an extra crispy crust: Add a teaspoon of cheese to the mini waffle maker for about 30 seconds before adding the recipe mixture. This will allow the cheese to get crispy when the tuna chaffle is done cooking. I prefer this method!

5. Add 1/2 the mixture to the waffle maker and cook it for a minimum of 4 minutes.
6. Remove it and cook the last tuna chaffle for another 4 minutes.

Nutrition:

Calories 320 Carbohydrates 2.9 g Protein 21.5 g Fat 24.3g

Blueberry & Brie Grilled Cheese Chaffle

Preparation time: 10 minutes

Cooking time: 10 minutes

Ingredients:

- 2 Chaffles
- 1 T Blueberry Compote
- 1 oz Wisconsin Brie sliced thin
- 1 T Kerrygold butter

Chaffle Ingredients:

- 1 egg, beaten
- 1/4 cup mozzarella shredded
- 1 tsp Swerve confectioners
- 1 T cream cheese softened
- 1/4 tsp baking powder
- 1/2 tsp vanilla extract

Blueberry Compote Ingredients:

- 1 cup blueberries washed

- Zest of 1/2 lemon
- 1 T lemon juice freshly squeezed
- 1 T Swerve Confectioners
- 1/8 tsp xanthan gum
- 2 T water

Directions:

1. Mix everything together.
2. Cook 1/2 batter for 2 1/2- 3 minutes in the mini waffle maker
3. Repeat.
4. Let cool slightly on a cooling rack.

Blueberry Compote Instructions:

5. Add everything except xanthan gum to a small saucepan. Bring to a boil, reduce heat and simmer for 5-10 minutes until it starts to thicken. Sprinkle with xanthan gum and stir well.
6. Remove from heat and let cool. Store in refrigerator until ready to use.

Grilled Cheese Instructions:

7. Heat butter in a small pan over medium heat. Place Brie slices on a Chaffle and top with generous 1 T scoop of prepared blueberry compote.
8. Place sandwich in pan and grill, flipping once until waffle is golden and cheese has melted, about 2 minutes per side.

Nutrition:

Calories 320 Carbohydrates 2.9 g Protein 21.5 g Fat 24.3g

BBQ Chicken Chaffle waffle

Preparation time: 3 minutes

Cooking time: 8 minutes

Servings: 2

Ingredients:

- 1/3 cup cooked chicken diced
- 1/2 cup shredded cheddar cheese
- 1 tbsp sugar-free bbq sauce
- 1 egg
- 1 tbsp almond flour

Directions:

1. Heat up your Dash mini waffle maker.
2. In a small bowl, mix the egg, almond flour, BBQ sauce, diced chicken, and Cheddar Cheese.
3. Add 1/2 of the batter into your mini waffle maker and cook for 4 minutes. If they are still a bit uncooked, leave it cooking for another 2 minutes. Then cook the rest of the batter to make a second chaffle.

4. Do not open the waffle maker before the 4 minute mark.

5. Enjoy alone or dip in BBQ Sauce or ranch dressing!

Nutrition:

Calories 320 Carbohydrates 2.9 g Protein 21.5 g Fat 24.3g

Cheddar Chicken and Broccoli Chaffle

Preparation time: 2 minutes

Cooking time: 8 minutes

Servings: 2

Ingredients:

- 1/4 cup cooked diced chicken
- 1/4 cup fresh broccoli chopped
- Shredded Cheddar cheese
- 1 egg
- 1/4 tsp garlic powder

Directions:

1. Heat up your Dash mini waffle maker.
2. In a small bowl, mix the egg, garlic powder, and cheddar cheese.
3. Add the broccoli and chicken and mix well.

4. Add 1/2 of the batter into your mini waffle maker and cook for 4 minutes. If they are still a bit uncooked, leave it cooking for another 2 minutes. Then cook the rest of the batter to make a second chaffle and then cook the third chaffle.

5. After cooking, remove from the pan and let sit for 2 minutes.

6. Dip in ranch dressing, sour cream, or enjoy alone.

Nutrition:

Calories 320 Carbohydrates 2.9 g Protein 21.5 g Fat 24.3g

Spinach & Artichoke Chicken Chaffle

Preparation time: 3 minutes

Cooking time: 8 minutes

Servings: 2

Ingredients:

- 1/3 cup cooked diced chicken
- 1/3 cup cooked spinach chopped
- 1/3 cup marinated artichokes chopped
- 1/3 cup shredded mozzarella cheese
- 1 ounce softened cream cheese
- 1/4 teaspoon garlic powder
- 1 egg

Directions:

1. Heat up your Dash mini waffle maker.
2. In a small bowl, mix the egg, garlic powder, cream cheese, and Mozzarella Cheese.

3. Add the spinach, artichoke, and chicken and mix well.
4. Add 1/3 of the batter into your mini waffle maker and cook for 4 minutes. If they are still a bit uncooked, leave it cooking for another 2 minutes. Then cook the rest of the batter to make a second chaffle and then cook the third chaffle.
5. After cooking, remove from the pan and let sit for 2 minutes.
6. Dip in ranch dressing, sour cream, or enjoy alone.

Nutrition:

Calories 320 Carbohydrates 2.9 g Protein 21.5 g Fat 24.3g

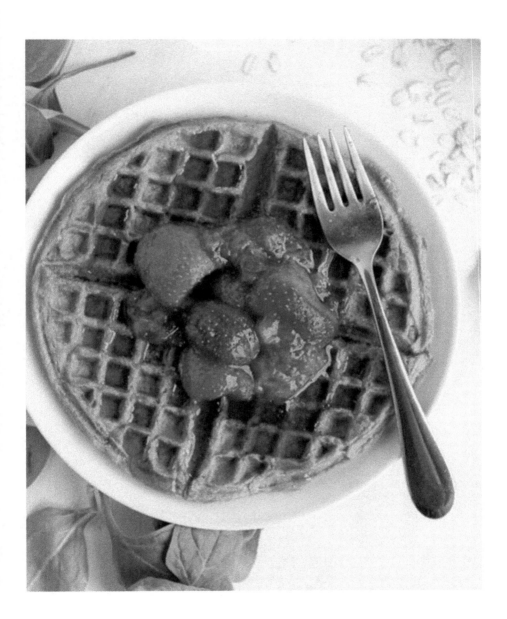

Lightning Source UK Ltd.
Milton Keynes UK
UKHW020628060521
383207UK00003B/285